STOP WRINKLES

THE EASY WAY

How to best care for
your skin and slow the
effects of ageing

**DR MIKE DILKES &
ALEXANDER ADAMS**

First published in Great Britain in 2021 by Orion Spring
an imprint of The Orion Publishing Group Ltd
Carmelite House, 50 Victoria Embankment
London EC4Y 0DZ

An Hachette UK Company

1 3 5 7 9 10 8 6 4 2

A CIP catalogue record for this book is
available from the British Library.

ISBN (Mass Market Paperback) 978 1 8418 8276 5
ISBN (eBook) 978 1 8418 8277 2

Printed and bound in Great Britain by
Clays Ltd, Elcograf, S.p.A

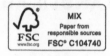

www.orionbooks.co.uk

ORION
SPRING

STOP
WRINKLES

Contents

1

The Basics of
Collagen and Elastin

To answer questions about wrinkles is really about understanding
the composition, nuances and physiology of the body's biggest
organ: the skin. Your skin makes up approximately 15 per cent of
your overall body weight, covering an area of 1.9 square metres
(21 square feet) and comprising 300 million skin cells, and home
to more than 1,000 species of bacteria at any given time.

The skin is a highly sophisticated organ with one key purpose:
to provide a barrier between the inside of the body and the
outside.[1] Providing a robust and permanent layer of protection
against physical aggressors, such as friction, chemicals and
infection, as well as harmful ultraviolet (UV) rays,[2] is, of course,
essential for the basic existence of human life. We define this
function as: skin the protector.

Since we are constantly exposed to billions of possibly infective
organisms it is quite humbling to recognise that the skin – despite

being thin and flexible – is an incredibly effective barrier and the main reason we aren't always ill. However, there are two further important functions of skin that we must understand. These are regulation and sensation.

Regulation

A much overused but accurate adage is to describe the skin as the body's thermostat because of its role in controlling the passage of water and electrolytes for the thermoregulation of the body. Receptors signal the need for shivering when one's core temperature drops below 36.9°C (98.42°F). Equally, if your body increases in temperature above 37.2°C (98.96°F), one of the 2–5 million sweat glands in the skin will instantly secrete sweat to cool the body down.

The skin is also responsible for regulating vitamin D levels. It acts as a reservoir lined with compounds that are catalysed using light and UV radiation into essential stores of vitamin D. This supports a properly functioning gut, bone density, cell growth, immune functions and reduces inflammation.[3]

Sensation

Skin sensations are broadly explained by three types: touch, hot and cold sensations, and, of course, pain. The sensation of touch begins with a very light impact that has no structural effect on the skin. Think of clothes touching the skin, which we are aware of but can mentally be put to one side throughout the day. If more pressure is applied to the skin, an ill-fitting belt buckle or watch perhaps, then the sensation becomes harder to ignore. The sensations of hot and cold, or pain, signal to the body that some things are a bad idea, like putting your hand in a fire! The skin therefore is primed to alarm you if the temperature dips below 20°C (68°F) or above 45°C (113°F) as this is the point where the skin begins to be damaged and we feel pain.

The Important Role of Collagen and Elastin

As we age, so too do we adopt an endless fascination with the firmness and tightness of our skin. Understanding the mechanisms of collagen and elastin is key to unlocking the secrets of wrinkle creation and prevention.

Collagen

This is the most abundant protein in the human body, accounting for around 30 per cent of its total protein content. It is formed by cells called fibroblasts among others. Collagen is the binding force around which connective tissue is formed, such as bone, ligaments and cartilage. It is the main structural protein in the skin and gives skin its firmness, in particular, resistance to trauma, such as pulling, tearing and penetration. Some diseases, such as Ehlers-Danloss syndrome, have defects in collagen, causing problems with skin (which becomes weak and easily deformed), ligaments (so joints are hypermobile) and blood vessels (where the blood vessel wall is weak and the pressure of blood within causes aneurysms (dilatations) to occur).

Elastin

This is elastic tissue, again a protein, that is made up of a combination of elastin protein and fibrillin protein, which are extensively cross-linked like a tight lattice that provides strength and flexibilty. It is particularly present in large blood vessels, which is why patients with the elastin defect known as Marfan's syndrome develop aortic aneurysms – a very serious condition of the biggest blood vessel in the body. Like collagen, Elastin is made by fibroblasts, but instead of increasing the firmness of the skin, it ensures the skin stays tight. It is also defective in some patients with emphysema of the lungs, due to overactivity of the enzyme elastase, which is caused by alpha-1 antitrypsin activity, such as inhaling smoke or other toxic materials like dust. Dermatochalasia is another condition caused by elastin insufficiency, in which the skin progressively hangs loose, leading to premature ageing. In addition, there is Geroderma osteodysplastica, or Walt Disney dwarf syndrome, which is also caused by elastin deficiency, and has premature ageing and sagging skin as one of its features.

Now that we understand the basic purpose of this multifunctional organ we can bring the composition of skin to life with a handy diagrammatic walk-through in the next chapter.

2

Skin Deep

The Anatomy of the Skin:
Explaining the Epidermis and the Dermis

Onions, humour and irony all have many layers, and so too does the skin. Getting to grips with these layers means that you will make better sense of the myriad of widely available facts and fiction on the topic of wrinkles. This will enable you to make an informed decision on how to correctly select and apply specific routines and remedies, in particular creams and drugs. More importantly it will help you understand when a wrinkle is, in fact, NOT a wrinkle and instead might be an indicator of more serious conditions.

Figure 1

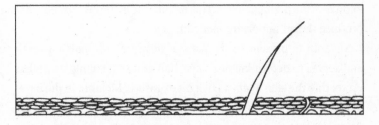

The cross-section above shows the primary layer of the skin, the layer we see, feel, cut, rub, sooth, sun-kiss and graze. This outer layer is the epidermis, which comes from the Latin *epi* meaning 'on' and *dermis* 'skin'. As described earlier this is the body's first line of defence, due to its ability to protect, regulate and give rise to sensations that signal the necessary response from the body.

Penetration of the epidermis is a significant cause of infection as the breaking of the skin means an open line of undefended entry. The outer skin is where you will see evidence of external forces manifested in rashes, blisters, sunspots and, of course . . . wrinkles

Figure 2

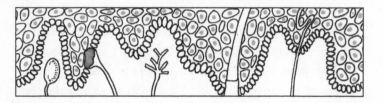

As we move down into the second layer we discover a fine strip of basal lamina which is the primary membrane, a boundary of living cells that sit below the skin and which is more commonly known as the pigment layer. This membrane contains the cells that produce the all-important melanin.

Melanin is present in the skin of nearly all animals on earth and serves to determine one's eye, hair and skin colour, as well as protecting the skin against UV light exposure. Melanin in the basal lamina absorbs UV light so it can't penetrate and damage deeper down. Lighter skin types have less melanin than darker skin types and therefore have less natural sun protection, therefore requiring more intervention in life. We will discuss this further in Chapter 5.

Figure 3

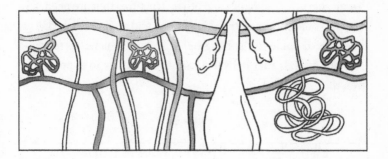

As fairer skin types have less protection it is easier for harmful UV rays to work their way through the epidermis and pigment layers into the next layer: the papillary dermis. For the purposes of this book this is perhaps the most important layer of the skin to understand for it is this layer that contains the two critical elements in the creation, prevention and reduction of wrinkles that we have already met: collagen and elastin.

Figure 4

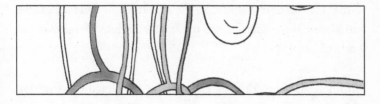

The fourth deep layer is the reticular dermis, which sits below the papillary dermis. This is a much thicker, denser layer that also contains collagen and elastin to give the skin further strength. Because it is deeper, it is less implicated in ageing and wrinkles as it doesn't get damaged by external forces, such as UV radiation. The reticular dermis contains sweat glands, sebum glands plus blood vessels, nerves, lymphatics and other structures that are needed to keep the outer layers of the skin healthy and well-nourished. This layer is also home to the large bulb-like hair follicles surrounded by blood vessels that deliver essential hormones to support hair growth.

Figure 5

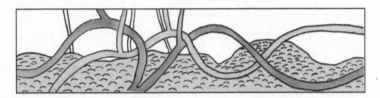

The final and deepest layer is a bed rock of fat – subcutaneous fat to be precise or the hypodermis. Primarily this zone protects the deeper structures of the body, in particular the muscles and the bones, but it's hugely important in the role of wrinkle treatment too. A good layer of fat 'plumps up' the skin, preventing any underlying sagging from becoming too prominent. 'Plumpness' is a much-used term to characterise youthful and aesthetically pleasing skin, so we will discuss this in more detail in Chapter 6 when we uncover the world of facial ageing.

Putting all this together we can see the completed cross-section of healthy skin, where all layers synchronise to play their own essential roles, and this illustrates the mechanisms at play in having tight and vigorous skin, the key to a youthful complexion.

Now that we broadly understand what the skin is and how it functions, we can begin to answer the question: 'So what causes wrinkles?'. In short, you're really asking: 'What actually is a wrinkle?'

Figure 6

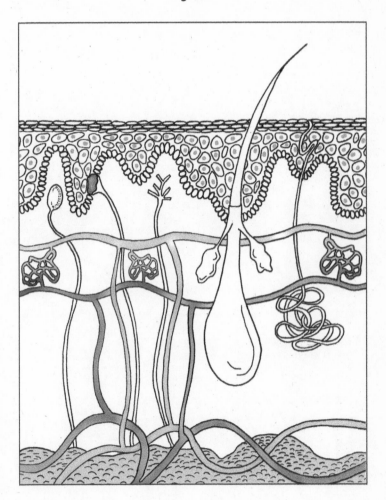

3

Understanding Wrinkles

What are Wrinkles?

Callum is five years old and for Christmas receives his dream gift – a brand-new trampoline. The next day he helps his father build the present in the back garden. It consists of a rigid outer frame, some firm stainless-steel springs and a large tightly woven and glossy net. Callum's father attaches each of the springs at half-metre intervals around the entirety of the outer frame. Once they have completed all but five springs the netting becomes increasingly rigid and more challenging to stretch and correctly align and place in the remaining loops. With some real force they stretch the remaining fabric enough to secure the loops and the trampoline is complete. The final stage is to cover the exposed mechanism, the springs, with a thick layer of padding, which attaches neatly into place.

If you have ever been on a trampoline, the first things you realise are just how hard the netting is, and the ease with which the huge pressures around the whole structure easily cope with your weight, flexing then snapping instantly back into place into its perfectly level and taut resting state. If you have ever been lucky enough to own a trampoline, then you will also know how neglected they are. They are almost always left out in the elements 100 per cent of the time, either used constantly or left unloved during the colder months of the year. Well-made models survive this treatment remarkably well and those that are well-maintained can last undamaged and in working order for years to come.

Callum is now sixteen and while his trampoline is still much loved, it is used more as an adolescent clubhouse than a toy. One late summer evening he and a few friends have taken to lazing on the netting and regaling each other about the events of the day. Eleven years prior the netting would barely have flexed under the weight of three children but after years of use and with the mass of three young adults, the material sags and rests with a pronounced slump in the centre, straining the loop fastenings and the springs.

When the boys eventually get up and leave for their respective dinner tables the netting does make every effort to return to its previously tight rested state but the continuous stretching has meant that the fibres of the net and, indeed the springs to which it's anchored, are no longer what they once were. It still functions exactly as it should, except for a slight reduction in spring, and is certainly in no way redundant, however, a number of visible indicators begin to show a steady decline in its overall integrity.

The centre of the net has lost a degree of stretch and appears ruffled somehow, more like a sail now rather than a tight net. In localised areas there are lighter patches were the net fibres have begun to fray and visibly fade in the heat of the summer. The most notable change, however, are the faint lines, almost creases, which run across the netting. Barely visible when pressure is applied but can be seen only in a resting state. As the years progress, these lines become deeper and more pronounced, and before long will completely change the composition of the net.

This example, while simple, provides the perfect lens through which to understand the process of decline in the human skin's structural integrity. The netting represents elastin; the springs, collagen; and the frame, the underlying skeletal structures.

'Decline' seems an overly harsh term to use here as it suggests there is nothing that can be done to reverse the process, and also that there is no hope, but as we shall discuss this could not be further from the truth. Perhaps 'natural process' is a less alarming phrase, but make no mistake that this continual journey of the skin is inevitable and it's how you acknowledge, prepare and respond that will have the biggest impact when trying to improve wrinkles.

As wrinkles on the trampoline emerge when sufficient and consistent pressure, strain or exposure occurs to the connective springs and netting, so too do wrinkles in the human skin. Remember, collagen makes the skin firm, and elastin makes the skin tight, so without protection a whole host of extrinsic factors attack the skin structures, slowly destroying the collagen and elastin fibres[4] and causing the skin's version of fault lines to begin to develop.[5]

Now let's take a look at why wrinkles appear on the skin. This is due to two key factors:

1. Environmental factors
2. Pressure memory

Environmental Factors

Sun exposure

It seems that we all know the sun is damaging to the skin and causes wrinkles. But beyond the throbbing evenings on sunburnt holidays, do we really understand the mechanism at work here? It is generally accepted that protecting the skin with sun-protection creams is beneficial both for longer-lasting aesthetic tanning and for preventing ageing of the skin. But why? Understanding this will hopefully make you think again if you are normally tempted to 'burn first' and then use creams on day two of your holiday!

Unless you are a honeybee, UV rays emitted from the sun are a light spectrum invisible to the eye. UV is a powerful force and supports everything from photosynthesis to generating essential vitamin D in the human body. This solar radiation is considered the most significant environmental factor affecting the skin, and the reason for this is because its contact with the skin generates free radicals – basically an atom that has become unstable. The skin is able to deal with a safe level of free radicals but once they exceed a certain point they begin to destroy cells, and in particular, elastin and collagen.[6] The breakdown of the tightness, firmness and the discoloration caused by UV radiation are the hallmarks of skin ageing.

Free radicals should be of much more concern than simply regarding one's appearance, as increased levels are also responsible for immunosuppression, a reduction in the body's immune system competence, the body's natural line of defence which opens us up to a host of far more serious and often life-threatening conditions. We will discuss this further in Chapter 5 when we outline some of the underlying conditions that wrinkles can be a symptom of.

A very popular term used by the health, nutrition and pharmaceutical industries that is linked to free radicals is 'antioxidant'. Much like 'superfood', antioxidants are something we 'know' have significant benefits, but in this case they are especially useful for skin health. This is because antioxidants are compounds that inhibit or block the process of formation of free radicals[7] and typically include vitamins, carotenoids and enzymes, which help form a protective layer in the skin and safeguard it from the destructive action of free radicals.[8]

Smoking

UV radiation is unavoidable but there are environmental factors, so called 'lifestyle' factors, affecting the skin that are entirely avoidable – most notably smoking.

Smoking has long been thought to speed up the natural ageing of the skin and is dependent on the length of time and quantity of cigarettes/cigars, etc. that you have been smoking. There are plenty of fresh-faced and blemish-free film stars smoking on the silver screen with little sign of these effects and the reason is simply their age. Wrinkles from smoking are most likely to appear after ten years of a pack a day and generally in the smoker's fourth decade. It is worth noting that even a pack a day pales in comparison to the effects of solar radiation (i.e. the sun's rays) on the skin, however, being exposed to both increases the process significantly, and – given the 6.5 trillion cigarettes that cater to 1 billion smokers worldwide[9] – the combination of smoking and UV light exposure is highly likely.

You might think that the issue here is the skin coming into contact with clouds of cigarette smoke, and while this contributes, the situation is actually internal and far more serious. Smoking nicotine causes a narrowing of the blood vessel that affects the proper blood flow and optimum condition of the skin, chronically depriving it of oxygen and nutrients.[10] With defences low, many of the 4,000 chemicals that make up a cigarette specifically target collagen and elastin – once again breaking down the strength and elasticity of the skin and causing sagging, which forms deep wrinkles and lines.

Smoking-related wrinkles are often part of the cause of facial ageing, however, it can be much worse than that. Elastin and collagen reside throughout the entire body and so will the damage caused by smoking. As such, current smokers might be concerned to hear that they will experience significant sagging in other areas too, namely the chest, neck, arms, midriff, etc. If you really care about the cosmetic effects of wrinkles and skin ageing, then smoking really is not an option at all. It is worth noting that alongside the aesthetic consequences of smoking, the more obvious reasons, such as lung disease, cancer and cost, should also serve as warnings against the habit.

Alcohol

It's often said that you 'can't out-train a bad diet', making clear that without proper nutrition, attaining that beach body or weight loss is near impossible to achieve. This extends to a host of other regimes and is a constant theme in the STOP series.[II] Diet is important for proper body function and relates closely to youthful and vibrant skin. As such, it is another environmental lifestyle condition to consider, especially as alcohol is so closely associated with smoking.

Firstly, social smoking while drinking alcohol is on the rise and the phrase, 'I only smoke when I drink' is the mainstay of those who visit pubs, bars and clubs, especially among those who abstain from buying their own cigarettes. Low use of cigarettes has far fewer implications than a pack a day, though; however, the breakdown of elastin and collagen is still underway even with moderate use. More importantly, alcohol depletes the body of vitamin A, which means your body is less well prepared to maintain healthy teeth, bones, soft tissues and, of course, skin.

This is not to say that you should immediately follow the advice from within the health and beauty industry that says the pursuit of the perfect complexion or body should trump the things in life, albeit vices, that make you happy. We are social creatures and shared events often make life worth living and should be enjoyed for the full function of mental health. 'You do you', as they say – however, it is important not to kid yourself. So, if you drink, smoke, bask in the sun and have a poor diet, the facts are that youthful and blemish-free skin is going to be impossible to achieve.

Low air humidity

Finally, in terms of environmental damage there is humidity – or, to be more specific, the quantity of water vapour in the atmosphere. Broadly, the range of humidity within the home varies around the world from 30 per cent to 60 per cent. Humidity is relative to temperature. For every 20°C (68°F) rise in temperature, the atmosphere roughly doubles its capacity to hold water vapour.

A recent study published in the *Journal of the European Academy of Dermatology and Venereology* reviewed the evidence on the effect that humidity has on both healthy and diseased skin.[12] The study found that even a 30 per cent difference in relative humidity[13] can affect skin properties in just thirty minutes. The authors found that a decrease in moisture levels led to decreases in the elasticity of the skin and a significant increase in fine wrinkles.

A moisture-rich climate also promotes rejuvenation of skin cells,[14] giving the skin a much brighter appearance, which is caused by the consequent reduction in dead cells on the skin's surface. The increased sweating that occurs in a more humid environment, much like after a hard run or workout, also makes the skin a good source of detoxification for the body as toxins can be secreted into sweat. Lack of moisture is key to the onset of signs of ageing, as we will discuss in Chapter 6. Ultimately any anti-ageing and wrinkle-reversal regime must include humidity and rehydration.

Pressure Memory

Environmental factors impacting the skin and resulting in wrinkles are perhaps the most understood by the general public. There is, however, a subset of actions that lead to wrinkles that you personally have much more control over – so we must now understand the world of pressure memory.

If we revisit the analogy of the trampoline, you will recall that one of the key factors in the appearance of fault lines in the netting was the consistent stretching over time – the netting fibres are used to being stretched and begin to remember the stretched state and adopt it as its resting state, thus causing wrinkles. This is what we mean by pressure memory and the skin works in exactly the same way. Facial wrinkles are often caused by pressure memory given the sheer number of expressions the surface of the face skin endures. However, there is one far more significant pressure that you have much more control over: the pressure caused by sleep.

A number of studies have proved the sheer amount of pressure that the body (in particular the head) exerts on the pillow and bedclothes at night. This pressure increases with certain neck and chin positions.[15] Sleeping position then has a huge impact on the pressure memory of the face and skin and the creation of wrinkles when one sleeps on the side of one's face or face down on the pillow each night. Sleeping on the side of your face pushes all the skeletal tissue upwards, or to one side depending on your sleeping position. It is essential that you understand the cumulative effect this has – guaranteeing that the pressure memory involved will cause the stretching of elastin over time, guaranteeing fault lines and wrinkles. The way to combat this is obviously to ensure restful sleep by sleeping on your back. This is easier said than done – and monitoring an optimum sleeping position while asleep is near impossible. So, for those that can't help but pass out face down, more consideration should be given to the pillows you use. This could protect you from the onset of early sleep-related ageing.

Sleep and sleep aids are a burgeoning industry, and there are pillows made from materials clinically proven to be less abrasive than standard-issue cotton and polyester. Silk pillows have been shown to reduce pressure-memory wrinkles, and a 2009 study showed that pillowcases that contain copper oxide not only considerably improved facial skin characteristics but can also rejuvenate the appearance of the face.[16] The study went on to conclude that consistent sleeping for four weeks on pillowcases containing copper oxide caused a significant reduction in the appearance of facial wrinkles and crow's feet/fine lines and contributed to a sizeable improvement in the overall appearance of facial skin. If it is a viable option for you, switching your pillowcase could make a positive difference.

4

Key Battle Grounds

Key Battlegrounds

Where do Wrinkles Appear?

Now that we understand how wrinkles are caused it is time to outline the problem areas. Facial wrinkles and fine lines are generally the area we focus on but it is useful to understand what we consider to be the three key wrinkle areas:

- Face
- Neck
- Chest

Face

Facial wrinkles and fine lines are the mainstay of cosmetics advertising and marketing campaigns, with countless methods to choose from in reducing the appearance of ageing on your 'moneymaker'. This is understandable as your face is literally the cover of your book, allowing onlookers to judge the many stories it can tell and the preconceptions about how one lives their life.

Worry and frown lines

Worry lines and frown lines are one of the first lines to appear on the face of men and women and are a result of the endless expressions that this section of the face is responsible for. The frontalis muscle of the forehead creases every time we frown, raise an eyebrow or emote.[17] Children will not yet develop these lines as they have no coarse eyebrow ridges and have prominent cheekbones[18] over which the skin is tightly stretched.

As we have described, the more the brow creases, the deeper the lines become and unless you plan to keep a completely expressionless face for your whole life, these are impossible to prevent. Worry lines are often more pronounced in men, especially as men are historically less likely to adopt a cosmetic regime to reduce and reverse the effects. This trend is changing, however, and the good news is, as we will outline in Chapter 6 that there are some highly effective measures that can be taken to mitigate the development of wrinkles.

Crow's feet

The periorbital region, from the Latin *peri*, meaning around or near, and *orbita*, meaning eye socket, is vulnerable to ageing. This area is defined by lines that run from the corners of the eyes in multiple strands often referred to as 'crow's feet'. The muscles in this area of the face are responsible for the movements of the eyelids[19] and are in near constant use.

Skin around the eyes is also at its most delicate on the face, so expressions, sun exposure and pollutants (like smoking) have a greater impact on the development of fine lines and wrinkles in this area. Anyone who has been skiing will remember the crow's feet tan lines on the faces of most après-ski revellers. Luckily these tan lines are temporary, but they give you some idea about the amount of time we spend squinting and moving the muscles around the eyes. Given the amount this region of the face is used, crow's feet are nearly impossible to avoid. However, the preventative science is increasingly robust and in Chapter 6 the methods that have shown aesthetic improvements as well as increases in collagen content and elasticity of the skin are outlined. For those of you panicking about the years spent squinting in the sun, you might find some comfort in the side note that a 2019 study showed that those people who had crow's feet were also likely to be very sincere, intense and positive.[20]

Smile lines

Smile lines develop ... you guessed it, from smiling. More specifically from the creasing of the skin at either side of the mouth. As the lips widen upon seeing a friendly face or hearing something particularly amusing, the lip raises too, ultimately meeting resistance with the soft tissues in the face and resulting in a fold. As the constant theme so far suggests, consistent flexing of this area, combined with a timely reduction in the integrity of elastin and collagen in the skin, means the folds leave faint lines and ultimately wrinkles or smile lines.

It is such a shame that the long-term act of something so positive and joyful (smiling) is associated with being unattractive or somehow undesirable in later life. Most of us would probably rather have a face that tells the story of a happy and fulfilled life, and yet we tend to peruse one that appears to have endured a bad smell at an endless poker game. That said it's well known that facial attractiveness (albeit subjective) plays a key role in social interaction.[21] We exist in a world that wants to have its cake and eat it; to conform to a standard of stereotypical beauty while having a life of laughter, revelry and being absorbed in the types of vices we have discussed seems an impossible dream. While the regimes in the second half of this book will teach you how to minimise and reverse the effects of smile lines, do recognise the cultural shift taking place across the world that rejects these frankly arcane standards of beauty.

Nasolabial lines

As we know, the skin loses its tightness over time due to a number of intrinsic and extrinsic processes causing a sagging of the skin, which leaves traces on the face in the form of wrinkles. Nasolabial lines are a clear indicator of ageing in the midface and run in line with the bridge of the nose down to the corners of the mouth, even as low as the jawline and over time extending to the outline of the cheeks. A little understood mechanism at work here is gravity. The cheeks are the most voluminous part of the face, and while supple and firm in one's early years, gravity forces the mass down, making nasolabial lines and folds more pronounced and once again tough to avoid.

Jawline and jowls

The effect of gravity is not limited to the midface and the cheeks. As we all get older the once sharp and chiselled jawline of one's youth also has its banks breached. This could simply be due to weight gain or significant weight loss over the years, but is also indicative of the muscle and soft tissue slowly slipping down the skeletal structures and causing a droop along the jawline. Interestingly, this is also because different parts of the body grow at different rates. The nasal system, for example, will not be at full size until the lungs are fully developed and in turn the body is developed enough to facilitate the full-grown breathing system.

As the structures of the face and body change, you are never really dealing with the same canvas as you were even a year before – and this should be taken into consideration in choosing (and your expectations of) a wrinkles' treatment programme.

Movements in teeth and the jawbone redefine the shape of the face on a near constant basis. Indeed this craniofacial growth continues long after young adulthood and into the later ages.[22] Perhaps you have developed an over- or underbite, which means your skin will over time become, in a sense, ill-fitting.

Neck

The conversation around wrinkles is dominated by issues relating to the face, but advances in rejuvenation treatments have meant more focus on additional areas where a breakdown of the skin's structural integrity results in skin folding, sagging and wrinkles. The neck is one such area and can tell you much more about the age of someone than can the deceptions of the face. As Nora Ephron writes in her standout essay *I Feel Bad About My Neck* 'Our faces are lies and our necks are the truth. You have to cut open a redwood tree to see how old it is, but you wouldn't if it had a neck'.[23]

Like the skin around the eyes, neck skin is very thin and is therefore far more susceptible to the effects of UV exposure, pollutants and gravity. Commonly observed aesthetic deficiencies of the neck include horizontal neck wrinkles, sagging of the skin with hanging folds, double chins and/or poorly defined jawlines.[24]

All the causes and effects discussed above of course apply to neck wrinkles too. However, a further contributing factor has become all the more relevant especially over the last fifteen years. Neck posture and resting position. In 2017, a town in the Netherlands took the drastic measure of installing colour-coded LED strips at pedestrian crossings at all traffic light locations. The hope is that they'll catch the eye of pedestrians who are too distracted by their smartphones to bother looking at the road, telling them when to cross and when not to cross by either glowing green or red, depending on the traffic light signals.[25] Not only is the need for this safety measure a slightly depressing insight but also an insight into the now common head position that at rest is cranked downwards is a major cause of skin sagging and folding and a primary cause of neck wrinkles.

Our posture and sedentary lives are such a concern that a 2019 study released an image of the work colleague of the future, in which the author William Higham describes the numerous health problems associated with a modern desk job.[26] This includes hunchbacks, red sore eyes and sagging neck skin. It is humbling to wonder if Higham knew just how pertinent his predictions were to become in the post-Covid-19 world for the millions of 'lockdown' employees working from home. Higham speaks of time spent in office chairs and at desks, features that might well be considered luxuries for many who now conduct business hunched over virtual meetings and classrooms from the 'office' bed and floor.

As we will discuss in Chapter 8 good treatments cannot outwork a poor lifestyle, and long-lasting wrinkle-reversal regimes *must* be supported by basic day-to-day routines in order to work at all. It is important now, more than ever, to act on this advice not just for the prevention wrinkles but for your holistic health and wellbeing.

Chest

Chest wrinkles sit firmly in the category of pressure-memory wrinkles and are most prevalent in women and are very difficult but not impossible to avoid. The pressure-memory mechanism comes predominantly from one's sleeping position. If you are lucky enough to be one of the 10 per cent of people that sleep on their back during the night, then the onset of chest wrinkles may never occur at all. However, if you are one of the 74 per cent that sleep on their side[27] chest wrinkles are a near certainty. The side position results in the lower half of the body being rigid at rest while the upper half is pushed downwards. Where the skin of the two halves meet you will find fine lines even in young adults and as the ageing process reduces the available elasticity, over time these fine lines will appear as wrinkles on the chest long term.

Quality of sleep is also a huge factor here as only 65 per cent of people say they get restful sleep three to four nights a week.[28] These levels are chronically low and prevent the body's natural process of stage 4 REM (rapid eye movement), sleep's mission to regenerate collagen and elastin, speeding up the effects of all wrinkles, in particular those on the chest.

Most studies on the subject suggest that we can bank the restorative sleep we all get at the weekend as Friday and then Saturday are the days where we sleep deeply the most. This backstop is quickly dwindling, however, especially in the city, where these nights are reserved primarily for social events and late nights (if not early mornings). There is a reason they call it 'beauty sleep' – without it you may always just be a pumpkin.

You might be thinking, why is it that women are more prone to chest wrinkles than men? Sleeping position and sleep quality surely apply equally to both. The second contributing factor is gravity and its effect on the breasts in females. Sagging occurs as the soft tissue is drawn downwards over time, causing a weakening or stretching of Cooper's ligaments[29] and overextending the skin on the chest.

Now that we understand what wrinkles are, and how and where they appear, it's important to outline the different skin types and the likelihood of how you personally are to get wrinkles and how seriously you need to adopt prevention as early as possible.

5

Skin Deeper

Skin Type

There are many skin types and the Fitzpatrick scale[30] provides a good indicator of how likely you are to form wrinkles in later life by categorising the amount of melanin in the skin across a scale of 1–6. The higher the number on the scale, the higher the amount of melanin, lessening the effect of UV rays on the skin and the onset of age-related wrinkles.

Skin type	Typical features	Tanning ability
1	Pale white skin	Always burns, does not tan
2	Fair skin	Burns easily, tans poorly
3	Darker white skin	Tans after initial burn
4	Light brown skin	Burns minimally, tans easily
5	Brown skin	Rarely burns, tans darkly easily
6	Dark brown or black skin	Never burns, always tans darkly

This is also a hugely important guide to which ethnic groups are most at risk of serious conditions, such as skin cancer and malignant melanomas. A quick glance at this tells us that the majority of cases are likely to be within skin types 1 and 2, and research estimates that 90 per cent of skin cancers are associated with sun exposure[31] and are most prevalent in Caucasian populations in regions, such as Australia and New Zealand.[32]

The scale also tells us that the highest rate of early-onset wrinkles will most likely be in Caucasian populations. Dark brown and black skin is a firm 6 on the skin types classification scale, suggesting a natural layer of protection akin to a SPF (sun protection factor) 30 sun cream. This means dark brown and black skin rarely burns and the UV breakdown of collagen is far less evident until the much later stages of life. While a clear complexion is a leading indicator of a healthy lifestyle it is essential that this does not cloud our judgement and neglect necessary precautions. While dark brown and black skin is less likely to elicit cosmetic concerns *everyone* must protect their skin.

The very real danger here is that the beauty industry drives the conversation towards white skin being affected much more than dark brown or black skin – which while true neglects to inform people with darker skin types that they are still at risk of skin cancer and melanoma and are therefore diagnosed at much later and more dangerous stages than Caucasian patients. A 2017 study showed that black people are four times more likely to be diagnosed with advanced-stage melanoma and tend to succumb at a rate of 1.5 times more than white people with a similar diagnosis.[33]

This results in a strange paradox. Those least likely to get skin cancer are also the most likely to die from it, which must serve as the harshest of reminders that the conversations around the pursuit of aesthetic improvements are complete nonsense if people are dying from preventable illnesses.

One thing the definitions from 1–6 above do not highlight are the further differences in skin type, such as those between males and females.

Male Versus Female Skin

Those of us who are not easily offended or who take criticism particularly well might be used to being described as having 'thick skin'. Whether or not you find this complimentary, the reality is this might actually have some truth to it. A number of studies have pointed towards the unique features between male and female skin and in particular those skin diseases that one gender can typically expect to have or avoid in their lifetimes.

Thicker skin is preferable as with thickness comes increases in our wrinkle-fighting friends elastin and collagen, as well as benefits, such as better sustained hydration and a more neutral PH. One study showed that the general thickness of all skin decreases over time, adding weight to the discussion earlier about wrinkle prevention becoming harder as you get older and lose natural tightness. Interestingly, the thickness of men's skin decreases from the age of twenty while women's skin remains broadly the same thickness until they are in their fifties.[34] Great news for women, right? Well, not exactly. Men have a few natural advantages when it comes to skin thickness; indeed they have a substantial head start. Men's skin is a whopping 25 per cent thicker than women's, so while the decreases in skin thickness will happen much later in the lives of females – males have 25 per cent extra skin to get through before the playing field is levelled.

In light of this it's worth stressing that men should take no less care in looking after their skin – but all being equal it is undeniable that most men will wrinkle at a later stage of life than women.

When is a Wrinkle Not Just a Wrinkle?

As mentioned, your skin, and often the face, is a litmus test for your overall health. Bags under the eyes or a grey complexion point towards lack of sleep, redness and burning to unprotected time in the sun and dry patches of skin indicate a lack of retained moisture and dryness. Wrinkles can, however, be evidence of processes at work far more serious than everyday concerns about ones complexion. One such example, born out of new research, suggests deep forehead lines can be a leading indicator of far more than simply memory lines from continued facial surprise.

Namely, forehead wrinkles could be a marker for cardiovascular disease. Atherosclerosis is the build-up of plaque in the arteries. Plaque restricts the proper flow of blood around the body and a full blockage will often result in heart attacks and strokes. The science behind the link between forehead wrinkles and cardiovascular health is that atherosclerosis has an oxidative effect on the collagen levels in the body.[35] As the blood vessels are so fine on the forehead and the skin there particularly thin, early signs of wrinkles in this area could point to a reduction in collagen rejuvenation and repair – and therefore a build-up of plaque in the arteries.

As terrifying as this sounds, the point here is to remind you that your primary concern must always be endorsing routines and regimes that support true health, performance and wellbeing. It is far too easy to err on the side of cosmetic perfection, but understanding what your body is telling you through the physical changes of your skin and face must come first.

6

The Daily 2's:
Part 1

Managing Expectations

We can all be fooled into thinking there is a magical solution to
our aesthetic failings and, as we will show you, there are some
genuinely extremely impactful measures you can take to prevent,
combat and reverse wrinkles. There is a significant BUT that we
must highlight, however. Most wrinkle warriors have a vision of
themselves as they once were – an aesthetic yardstick to which
they must cling and return to at (literally) any cost. As we have
discussed above, ageing is not just about wrinkles; if this were
true, it would follow that if you removed the wrinkles of a sixty-
five-year man or women, instantly the face of their twenty-year-old
self would reappear. But, as you should now understand, facial
ageing involves structural changes to both the face and the body,
so it is worth bearing in mind the following statement to manage
your expectations.

If you were once a grape but now find yourself to be a raisin, even a complete reversal of wrinkles and rebuild of skin elasticity and collagen would not return you to your former golden grape days. Rather you will be a perfectly wrinkle-free raisin (a stunning sultana at best).

How Do I Stop Wrinkles from Forming?

Having read the earlier chapters, you will know that there are primary causes of wrinkles. We have therefore outlined a set of easy to adopt, daily best practices to stop wrinkles in their tracks and prevent them altogether. The great thing about the basics is that they are something you can easily implement immediately and are mostly free or, at most, inexpensive.

Below is a checklist that you can remember and deploy every day. Just ask yourself: Have I done the 2s?

The Daily 2s

- 2 litres of water
- 2 portions of good bacteria and collagen
- 2 applications of SPF 30
- 2-minute face cleanse
- Off 2 sleep (sleep hygiene and sleep quality)

This checklist is fully explained below and includes ways that you can go above and beyond to maximise results. Pre-empting an almost inevitable sigh – the fact is that what you put into your body is essential to ensure vibrant and collagen-filled skin long-term. Much as you can't out-train a bad diet, you can't naturally un-wrinkle poorly maintained skin. In this chapter we will outline the first three actions on the daily 2s checklist. They are easy and straightforward, and you can put them into action today.

Two Litres of Water

Two litres of water a day is the absolute bare minimum you must drink. And don't be thinking you can supplement with teas, coffees, juices, smoothies or cocktails. Telling you to stop all poor hydration choices is a pointless (and unnecessary) exercise, but the point is if you choose to drink high-fructose or alcoholic drinks, that's fine, although a reduction will maximise your results, but you can't miss out the water on top. No ifs and no buts.

Proper hydration supports key bodily functions and keeps your body in full working order, as well as giving a host of benefits, such as helping the skin correctly regulate temperature, maintain optimum blood pressure and lubricate joints. It also prevents the early breakdown of elastin. Those who are well hydrated also benefit from supple-looking and plump skin, especially on the face, which we know reduces the appearance of wrinkles.

Drink more and quit caffeine

Now that you have added base-level hydration to your day, you might be asking 'How can I take this further?' Great question. Simple answer? Drink more and cut out the caffeine. The reality is that two litres is really not a huge amount, especially if you work out regularly. Maintaining the two litres alone will have huge effects on your whole-body health, but the more you increase the amount, the bigger positive effect there will be on your health, wellbeing, anxiety levels and, of course, your complexion. Indeed the results can be so significant, one experiment showed that increasing your daily water intake to three litres can shave ten years off one's appearance with significant results shown within two weeks.[36]

As with most things it seems the simplest solutions are often the most effective and the good news is that the results multiply again if you take the bold step to knock caffeine on the head too. This might seem like the unimaginable and for the many patients we speak to – as well as the 83 per cent of adults who drink coffee every day[37] – the ritual morning craving for an aromatic pick-me-up is near impossible to forgo. But what if we were to tell you that caffeine is what is making you tired and giving you wrinkles? Would you think again?

We have already established that hydration is everything, so in the pursuit of the perfect complexion it seems counter-intuitive to rely on drinks (teas, coffees, cold brews, energy drinks, etc.) that actively dehydrate, not to mention the stress they put on the body through increased heart rate and elevated blood pressure. Ironically, your morning cup of joe is the reason you need a second, third and fourth cup throughout the day, as the artificial energy spike you gain in the short term (along with the jitters and anxiety) needs to be maintained to avoid a crash. As with any other drug we also build up a tolerance to the effects and, before you know it, you are measuring consumption by the pot, not just the mug. Most importantly, the crashes continue into the night, preventing reliable REM sleep, the only time when your body can rebuild and replenish its stores of elastin and collagen.

The bad news is that quitting caffeine does come with two to three days of sometimes harsh withdrawals, and that in itself is a valuable sign for you to consider what you're putting in your body. After the three-day hump, though, amazing things begin to happen – most notably the effects of proper restful and regenerative sleep.

The best course of action therefore is to replace your morning tea or coffee with hot water. Lemon, honey or ginger can make this a more aromatic experience if that mental trigger is something you still rely on. This might seem like an extreme step but it is essential in the pursuit and maintenance of inexpensive and highly effective wrinkle-reducing results – and we hear all the time that after the first few days the hot water substitute provides exactly the routine you had before, plus the two coffees a day you're no longer buying from the local coffee house is now saving you over £2,000 a year. Just saying.

Two Portions of Good Bacteria and Dietary Collagen

The father of medicine, Hippocrates, famously declared that 'all disease begins in the gut',[38] pointing to the fact that poor gut health and insufficient 'good bacteria' has huge implications for our overall health, and therefore our skin quality, which reminds us again that 'beauty comes from within'.

Good bacteria

The two portions of good bacteria are designed to go much further than standard healthy balanced diet advice – although this is, of course, very important. Remember your face, chest and neck wrinkles are the visual evidence of how you spend your life and a key indicator of your overall diet. It is not the job of this book to warn you about meat-based, vegetarian or vegan meals that are overly processed. This is most probably nothing new to you and the literature on this topic is conclusive. The key departure here is that for optimum skin health, and the prevention and reduction in wrinkle depth, you must incorporate an item of good bacteria into your diet in at least two of your meals daily.

Foods commonly associated with gut health come under the umbrella of 'fermented'. Fermented foods contain a wealth of essential and beneficial bacteria that support a healthy gut or 'microbiome'.[39] It is only in recent years that the full extent of how important the microbiome truly is to our overall health – including the brain, digestion and immune system, along with the cosmetic features of the body's outermost surfaces – has come to light.

The simple routine is to have two portions of fermented whole foods each day. The easiest way to do this is by incorporating them into your existing meal plan. For example, salmon fillets, rice, leafy greens and a side of kimchi, a fermented Korean spicy cabbage. Or a breakfast bowl of fruit, berries, seeds and Kefir, a fermented milk-derived probiotic yogurt, which is also 99 per cent lactose-free[40] and a great addition to cereals, smoothies and protein shakes. The full list for you to choose your two a day from is:

- Kimchi
- Kefir
- Miso (a paste made of fermented soya beans, often found in soup)
- Sauerkraut (finely chopped fermented cabbage)
- Sourdough (bread that is far easier to digest and made from fermented dough)
- Kombucha (fermented tea)

There are also a host of additional food stuffs that good bacteria enjoy and which are easily added to your daily meals. These are not fermented but play an essential role in good gut health and are most likely foods you already have at home:

- Extra-virgin olive oil
- Almonds
- Bananas
- Garlic (not just a vampire killer, garlic is also a powerful wrinkle-killer)
- Ginger (which you may already be adding to your morning hot water)

Dietary collagen

As you will recall from Chapter 1, collagen is the most abundant protein in the human body and is responsible for the structure, stability and strength of the skin.[41] The breakdown of collagen is a significant cause of the deterioration of skin health and therefore undesirable wrinkles. Enhancing stores of collagen in the body has been shown to improve the appearance and depth of wrinkles, especially on the face and neck. In a series of studies from 2006 to 2018 it was found that ingesting collagen consistently resulted in significant increases in both the diameter and density of collagen fibres,[42] but also that ingesting 7 grams of commercially available collagen daily increased the moisture content of the face, neck, forearm and chest, and led to major improvements in the pliability and elasticity of the skin, resulting in greater smoothness and . . . a reduction in wrinkles.[43]

Consuming daily collagen is essential to the daily 2s and, as is always our advice, wherever possible you should get your daily dose from nutritionally rich whole foods. Add two portions of the following to your meals without fail for maximum wrinkle reduction:

- Beef
- Chicken
- Fish
- Beans or legumes
- Eggs
- Dairy products

Bone broths are unimaginably effective as they make use of the full nutritional value of the meat and the vital collagen stores held within the bones and bone marrow. While not a whole food you could also get your daily collagen from a supplement powder added to a shake or mixed into a meal. It's also important to remember that optimum intake of collagen is supported by your intake of other essential vitamins, especially vitamin C, so ensure your meals also regularly incorporate:

- Raw or steamed leafy greens
- Citrus fruits
- Red and green peppers
- Steamed, raw or baked broccoli

Dairy, bad news for vegetarians and vegans?

Until very recently collagen sources with high bioavailability (in other words a source that has any meaningful result) could only come from animal products. A number of products have been released that use synthesised plant-based collagens, but it must be stressed that these are not dietary products; they are topical creams. The reality is that vegans and vegetarians will struggle to supplement and benefit from any dietary collagen at all. It is also worth noting that these groups must take particular care in the quality of the food they eat due to the negative effects of the standard vegan/vegetarian diet and the highly refined grains, starches, processed meat substitutes and high wheat and sugar contents they contain.[44]

Remember, beauty comes from within, so diets that stray from clean whole foods consistently show negative health and beauty signals, such as sagging, dry and dull skin, hair and nails and, of course, wrinkles. Vegans and vegetarians should take extra care to follow the other elements of the daily 2s and increase water and fermented food intake to three.

Two Applications of Factor 30

The Fitzpatrick Skin Type Classification scale showed us that not all skins are created equal but highlighted the importance of following the same skin-protection regime no matter your skin type. We also know that it does not have to be summer, or even sunny weather, in order for wrinkle-causing UV rays to damage the skin.

The market is flooded with thousands of different creams reporting to do everything from 'rebuilding collagen and elastin' to 'turning back the hands of time'. Undoubtedly, these creams, lotions and ointments can be highly effective, but the sheer choice is impossible to navigate. So we are going to make this really simple. For the best results in preventing the formation of and reduction in the depth of face, neck and chest wrinkles you need to choose a single cream that contains three essential elements and nothing more:

• Quality moisturiser
• Mineral-dense SPF 30
• Vitamin E

A high-quality moisturiser does just that. They are water-based or aqueous creams that maintain the moisture levels of the skin throughout the day by holding water on the skin surface, resulting in a plump and full complexion and, critically, softening hard lines and reducing wrinkle depth. This alone is an essential step, but if you use a cream that contains an SPF of at least 30, the results increase significantly once again.

The ingredients in creams that provide UV protection are chemical filters that prevent harmful pollutants and rays interacting negatively with the skin. With skin cancer diagnosis on the rise[45] the world's health organisations have quite rightly advised that all sunscreens are safe to use as there is overwhelming evidence that they protect the skin against cancer[46] and we wholeheartedly agree.

When it comes to UV protection and wrinkles, however, there is one important factor to consider when choosing your cream for the daily 2s. Sun protection in sunscreen is provided by chemical filters, such as oxybenzone or avobenzone, but there are also creams available that use mineral filters instead and it is the creams with the latter that we urge you to use. Mineral filters, such as zinc oxide or titanium oxide, are the only filters that are generally recognised as safe and effective to use. Mineral filters protect the skin from UV and do not damage the skin in and of itself. Chemical filters, on the other hand, block the UV rays but also penetrate the skin, causing damage to the dermal layers[47] and, ironically, can break down the essential elastic structure and cause wrinkles. Therefore, for full UV and cosmetic protection, you must choose an SPF moisturiser containing mineral (sometimes referred to as 'physical') filters only.

To complete the Holy Trinity of the ultimate daily 2 cream you must include the near magic ingredient Vitamin E. This vitamin is an important and powerful antioxidant that has been in use for more than fifty years in dermatology.[48] Its use is implicated in many areas of skincare from curing eczema, reversing sagging skin and, more importantly, skin ageing. The reason that we include it here, however, is that Vitamin E is able to mop up a host of free radicals that otherwise damage the skin. As more and more people live in increasingly urban areas, this provides good-quality protection against common airborne city pollutants that the vast majority of people will unknowingly be in contact with.

A Note on Peels, Hydra facials and Botox

For most of us naturally healthy-looking skin is the ideal goal, and the beauty of the daily 2s is that this is exactly what you can expect without resorting to time in the doctor's chair or under the knife. There are a growing number of medical procedures that do not promote a natural complexion and therefore are not procedures we recommend in this book. Nor are we in favour of interventions that promote an unrealistic body and beauty image and reliably unreliable results. There are three skincare procedures we did want to touch on briefly, though, as they are now common high-street options. Please note that if you were to choose or have chosen these procedures in the past, the baseline is to ensure you commit to the daily 2s, as this is the proven way for natural and consistent results. A quick fix sounds great, but, as we will discuss, it's never that straightforward.

Face peels, not to be confused with hydrating face masks, come in a number of guises, the most popular (and the mildest) is the fruit-acid face peel and can be administered by a beauty therapist or, slightly alarmingly, in a DIY home kit. These kits are safe to use at home, but we would highly recommend that anything acid-based is administered by a professional in the first few instances. You can then take their advice on which DIY kit is safe and best suited to your skin.

Peels are water soluble, so only affect the superficial layers of the skin, causing a mild inflammation, which then removes dead skin, exfoliates and speeds up cell turnover.[49] In reality, the effect the peels have on the reduction of wrinkles is inconclusive and, while generating new cells is no bad thing, there is no relation between exfoliation and the repair or maintenance of collagen or elastin. This type of practice is designed for those with skin conditions, such acne, scarring or uneven skin tone, for which they can be highly effective.

The story is slightly different, however, for the HydraFacials, a four-step non-invasive procedure that involves cleansing, exfoliating, extracting and hydrating the skin with serums that are infused into pores with a pen-like device.[50] In effect, the fine jets of serum are a detox for the face – removing blackheads and unblocking pores and replacing them with moisturising additives. While not a cheap procedure the results are consistent in that patients will see a more plump, bright and hydrated complexion, all of which will reduce the appearance of wrinkles. Once again, choosing this procedure must be as well as, and not instead of, a daily commitment to the daily 2s, and is only suitable for those wanting to reduce not prevent wrinkles.

Finally, the use of injectable substances to treat skin, in particular lines on the face, has increased almost exponentially over the past twenty years. The most common agent for this is Botox, which is essentially a toxin from the bacterium Clostridium botulinum. In the old days, to have botulism was to be poisoned and need immediate medical treatment, often a near death or indeed deadly experience. Nowadays it's one of the most common 'beauty'-enhancing treatments out there. It works because the toxin (called a neurotoxin) binds to a junction between a nerve and a muscle. This causes the muscle to be unable to move or contract, so it loses all its power and tone, causing skin to relax and lines to flatten out. Lines that are caused by active movement – such as frown and forehead lines and crow's feet are most affected. Contrary to popular belief it doesn't work for sagging skin that has lost its tone, and although it does work well around the mouth, it would be far too likely to cause drooling so is used sparingly in this area.

Botox is considered a reactive rather than preventative tool; however, some younger people do use it to stop lines forming in the first place, again, especially with crow's feet and forehead and frown lines, as stopping these areas moving and therefore the skin from creasing, prevents lines from forming.

Botox does also wear off after three to four months. This is because new receptors form in the junction between nerve and muscle, so the muscle starts to move again, and therefore the treatment has to be repeated. Botox treatments are not cheap and once you have started it's very difficult to stop as the results fade.

As with most unnatural remedies there is often a short-term gain and long-term loss, and this is important to remember if you are considering a treatment of this kind.

The final instalments of the daily 2s, while just as simple as those prior are best explained separately. As such, in chapters 7 and 8 we move on to outline:

- 2-minute face cleanse
- Off 2 sleep

7

The Daily 2's:
Part 2

Two-minute Face Cleanse

Useful advice and methods of correctly applying creams are now popular and widely available, so much so that it seems like going over old ground to reiterate them here. What is clear, however, is that it is not so much about *what* you put on your skin (although this helps, of course). Far more underestimated is what you are taking off – or, rather, how you are taking it off – in particular the night-time routines of many women and men that involve continued abrasive interactions with the skin. It has always been baffling to see the care at which people take in applying skincare products while having little to no concern about the heavy rubbing of the face and pulling and stretching the skin from left to right. Or indeed the number of stripping and removal lotions administered with piping-hot water and often coarse flannels and pads. As outlined in Chapter 3, these routines are pressure memory 101 and are far more likely to give you wrinkles than the latest wonder cream is to reverse them.

Removing make-up, washing the face and applying creams should all follow the same non-abrasive and low-impact formula to prevent the effects of pressure memory while at the same time stimulating the dermis and supporting collagen and elastin regeneration.

To make this really simple Figure 7 below separates the face into quadrants:

- Upper left
- Upper right
- Lower left
- Lower right

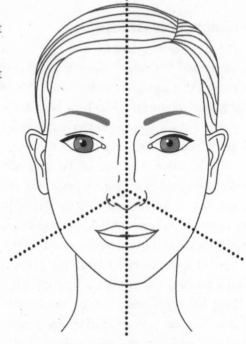

Figure 7

The golden rule is to attend to each quadrant separately with smooth movements, starting from the centre and moving outwards. The ensures minimal adverse pressure memory.

The two upper quadrants are slightly bigger than the lower two. This is due to the delicate skin around the eye and to keep the cleaning motions in line with the natural contours of the cheekbones, but the message is the same for all quadrants: 'wipe DON'T rub'. Taking upper left in isolation let's make this method really clear.

After rinsing the face with lukewarm (but ideally cold) water, using a pad or microfibre flannel, draw from the nostril and along the top boundary of the nasolabial fold as shown above. Then work upwards, taking particular care to move in the same direction at all times, rather than going back and forth. The area under the eye is where the skin is at its most delicate and susceptible to pressure memory and it is tempting be rough especially if there is mascara on the upper and lower eyelids. Remember, rubbing the skin is undoing all the good work done by the correct cream choice so

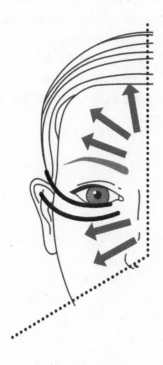

Figure 8

you must be patient when properly cleansing this part of the eye. Continue with the same motions for all other quadrants. Once you have done this a few times it should take no longer than two minutes from start to finish.

This method is optimal at removing make-up without promoting pressure memory and the early onset of wrinkles, but a 2017 study showed that massaging the skin in this way has a second essential mechanism in influencing cell behaviour and increasing the proteins and stiffness of the skin. The study assessed the key problem areas of facial wrinkles, skin texture, lip area, cheek wrinkles, neck sagging and neck texture and found that massaging the skin evoked a clear anti-ageing response which amplified the beneficial effects of night and day face creams.[51]

The dual-action cleanse is one of the most powerful tools you have in preventing and reversing the effects of facial and neck wrinkles and asks nothing more than that patients master the 'wipe NOT rub' philosophy.

8

Beauty Sleep

Off 2 Sleep

Now for the last of the daily 2s. Truly understanding the importance of sleep is a constant theme in health, wealth and nutrition literature, so it's no surprise that restorative sleep is just as important for one's cosmetic appearance.

The regenerative phases of sleep – stage 4 deep sleep and REM sleep – are all too absent in many adults across the age range, given the modern requirements of the workplace and sources of endless entertainment at night. These all combine to prevent sufficient sleep time and are chronically deficient among the world's insomniacs and snorers. Inability to enter regular regenerative sleep means the body is unable to repair collagen and in itself results in unhealthy, grey, loose and lined skin. As we have discussed, creams, procedures and routines can have a significant effect in reducing and removing wrinkles but there is a major caveat that is much under appreciated. The efficacy of the daily 2s will only sustainably work if you allow your body the basic protection it needs to work effectively. You can't do without sleep.

Proper Sleep Hygiene

The first step towards sleeping better is to consider your sleep hygiene. The term 'hygiene' brings to mind a focus on personal cleanliness prior to bed, maybe fresh bedding or an ordered, clutter-free bedroom. While these elements would help ensure a better night's rest in a practical sense, it's actually what they contribute to that defines what is meant by proper sleep hygiene: a routine that prepares us mentally for healthy sleep and daytime alertness.

One key observation we have made is that rather than seeing our bed as a place for rest, it is more commonly an extension of the living space. Watching TV and movies, playing games, reading and eating are now very normal activities that take place in the bedroom and this needs to change.

We understand that following the daily 2s thus far may already involve a significant behavioural change and lumping more change on top may tip the balance in favour of failure. Therefore, we have created a blue print for good sleep and ask that you incorporate the advice points as and when you are able, slowly making them a habit. Before you know it, they will be part of how you set up your day and night, and you'll be reaping the benefits in your overall health and skin health very quickly – guaranteed.

Blueprint for Good Sleep Hygiene

This list is by no means exhaustive but highlights some key first steps in getting sleep hygiene right. The idea here is to redefine the bedroom as a place we associate predominantly with sleep.

1. Don't eat high-calorie meals close to bedtime and be aware of what is in your snacks and evening treats, for example, chocolate contains caffeine.

2. Cut out stimulants, such as tea and coffee[52], ideally entirely but failing that, at least two to three hours prior to bed.

3. Try to avoid strenuous exercise in the evening and carry it out in the morning or afternoon instead.

4. Get outside in the day! Maximising your exposure to natural light will help regulate your internal body clock.

5. Don't nap in the day, even if you're tired. Get the regime right and you will see a rise in your energy levels so midday napping becomes a thing of the past.

6. Turn off all laptops, TVs, radios and close this book at least one hour before sleep. Mental stimulation will prevent you from entering restorative sleep.

One major change to people's lives due to COVID-19 (and some might suggest benefit of), COVID-19 has been the reduction in the amount of time many spend commuting to and from work every day. While we are hopeful of a speedy return, on the whole, to working as we knew it before the pandemic, this does provide a real and unique opportunity to ensure the real adoption of the best practices outlined earlier.

For most, the thought of an extra hour in bed is a comforting thought but can lead to later bedtime hours the night before. Please try to resist the urge to become a night owl. Proper REM sleep is one of the most powerful tools you have for both natural wrinkle-fighting and also in supporting your mental wellbeing with much needed rest.

One suggestion we would make, if you dare, is to turn off the alarm clock. The extra time you have in the morning is ideal to test and perfect waking up naturally, with the body clock alone. Alarm clock anxiety, the impending fear that the time to get up is creeping ever closer is a major cause of being unable to fall asleep at night.

It can start your day with a critical dose of cortisol, the stress hormone, as the day break ringing jolts you awake, which over time can cause high heart rates and most concerningly, high blood pressure. Start at weekends if you worry you will over sleep, but we guarantee you will eventually be waking up naturally, often earlier than your original alarm clear-headed, rested and stress-free.

While seemingly the easiest of the daily 2s, off 2 sleep is actually something you must work at, to undo many of the deep-rooted behaviours holding you back. The best advice is to adopt two of the sleep blueprint actions each week and restfully ease yourself into new sleep-enduing habits.

9

Give Blood

Before we conclude this guide to stopping wrinkles the easy way, there is one more action to consider. The final action is not one of the daily 2s but could become something you volunteer to do once or twice a year and, as well as having wrinkle-reversing benefits, will have a guaranteed impact on the wellbeing of society as a whole.

Giving Blood and Pumping Iron for Real

Giving blood can often literally mean giving another human being the gift of life. Anyone can give and few too many actually do. Blood is the lifeline for many who find themselves in an emergency or those that need long-term care. If you found yourself in need of blood, you would accept it in a second, and this is why it is so important that you offer this essential service in return. But why are we talking about helping others? Isn't this book meant to be all about you and your daily battle with ageing?

The body demands numerous vitamins and minerals that are essential to our growth and development from childhood to adulthood. One of the most essential minerals in this process is iron. It is found most abundantly in red meat, poultry and fish (but also in leafy greens and dried fruits) and is utilised by the body to create haemoglobin, which carries oxygen from the lungs throughout the body as red blood cells.

Iron is not all positive, however. Yes, it provides an essential service to the body, but it is still a highly reactive metal that can cause serious damage if not flushed through the body correctly. A healthy woman is able to purge her system of iron through her monthly menstrual cycles, expelling excess blood and keeping her iron levels to a productive and healthy level. Post-menopausal women, and men are not able to expel iron in the same way and, as a result, the levels of iron in the body rise, including within the skin.[53] This is a very slow process, but eventually the excess iron will create oxidation that can stress the functions and structures of our skin cells[54] and . . . create wrinkles.

But if this oxidative damage worsens, then wrinkles are probably not in the forefront of your mind given the effects this can have on the liver, brain, muscle and kidneys.

There is, of course, a wealth of research that shows those with excess iron, simple dietary adjustments that naturally flush the system, which, as luck would have it, are the very same supplements already recommended in this book. In particular, the uses of specific antioxidants, including turmeric, green tea and our good friend Vitamin E, are beneficial.

Yet there is a by far more powerful way to rid the body of iron build-up and prevent wrinkles caused by skin damage – giving blood!

P. D. Mangan's thesis 'Dumping Iron: How to Ditch This Secret Killer and Reclaim Your Health' shows that the most effective way of ensuring individual and social wellbeing is regular blood donation, which moreover serves as one of the most novel and simple approaches to premature ageing of the skin.

However, 90 per cent of those eligible to give blood never do despite the fact that in under an hour of painless time, you could save lives and improve your own health. The general guidance is that men can donate four times a year and women three times a year up to a threshold age of seventy.

If you can, give blood. It's great for you and it's great for society.

Conclusion

We hope this book has helped you make better sense of what wrinkles are (and indeed what they aren't) and shown how you can effectively take the actions needed to reduce and prevent them. We have tried to shift the indelible reputation that wrinkles are an inevitable 'will have' to a positive 'needn't have'. It may be true that some are more prone to wrinkles than others and some will have a tougher battle to prevent and repair them, but the fact remains that the mechanisms that cause wrinkles to appear are the same for us all.

Anyone, indeed everyone, can now identify those behaviours that are the root causes of *their* wrinkles and adopt some simple daily changes that will have the biggest impact. We've learned that wrinkles serve as one of the leading indicators of strains and stresses throughout the body as a whole. We know that cosmetic concerns will broadly be the reason you decide to act, but it's important to remember that this should be about making changes to support your holistic health and wellbeing, which just happen to have some amazing effects on your skin too.

Making the most of this guide requires an assessment of how you live your life and, we hope, a true appraisal of what's really important to you. Taking ownership of your health and combating wrinkles is not just about you and has wide-reaching effects for society as a whole. Eating higher-quality foods, financial savings, increasing your energy and positivity are all benefits that extend far beyond ourselves and something we hope you will join us in promoting around the world. We wish you all the very best success with this guide and are confident that you will join the thousands who have managed to STOP THE EASY WAY!

References

1 M. A. Farage, K. W. Miller, P. Elsner and H. I. Maibach,
'Characteristics of the Aging Skin', *Adv Wound Care (New Rochelle)*, February 2013, volume 2, issue 1, pp. 5–10

2 See www.bepanthen.co.uk/en/understanding-your-skin/your-skins-structure

3 See ods.od.nih.gov/factsheets/VitaminD-HealthProfessional

4 S. A. Monteiro, B. Michniak-Kohn and G. Leonardi, 'An overview about oxidation in clinical practice of skin aging', *Anais Brasileiros de Dermatologia*, 2017, volume 92, pp. 367–74

5 Goesel Anson, Michael A. C. Kane and Val Lambros, 'Sleep Wrinkles: Facial Aging and Facial Distortion During Sleep', *Aesthetic Surgery Journal*, September 2016, volume 36, issue 8, pp. 931–40

6 M. E. Darvin, H. Richter, S. Ahlberg, S. F. Haag, M. C. Meinke, D. Le Quintrec, O. Doucet, J. Lademann, 'Influence of sun exposure on the cutaneous collagen/elastin fibers and carotenoids: negative effects can be reduced by application of sunscreen', *Journal of Biophotonics*, 2014, volume 7, issue 9, pp. 735–743

7   S. A. Monteiroe Silva, B. Michniak-Kohn and G. R. Leonardi, 'An overview about oxidation in clinical practice of skin aging', *Anais Brasileiros de Dermatologia*, 2017, volume 92, pp. 367–74

8   Ibid. pp. 735–743

9   See www.verywellmind.com/global-smoking-statistics-for-2002-2824393

10 See www.webmd.com/smoking-cessation/ss/slideshow-ways-smoking-affects-looks

11 See the other books in our series: *Stop Snoring* and *Stop Allergies*

12 See www.skinhealthalliance.org/news/could-humidity-hold-the-key-to-looking-younger

13 Relative humidity (RH) is the most common way of measuring the moisture of the air.

14 See www.edit.sundayriley.com/how-does-humidity-affect-skin

15 B. Atwater, E. Wahrenbrock, J. Benumof and W. Mazzei, 'Pressure on the Face While in the Prone Position: ProneView Versus Prone Positioner', *Journal of Clinical Anesthesia*, March 2004, volume 16, issue 2, pp. 111–116

16 G. Borkow, J. Gabbay, A. Lyakhovitsky and M. Huszar, 'Improvement of facial skin characteristics using copper oxide containing pillowcases: a double-blind, placebo-controlled, parallel, randomized study, *International Journal of Cosmetic Science*, October 2009, volume 31, issue 6, pp. 437–443

17 See www.fatherly.com/health-science/forehead-wrinkles-treatments-for-men

18 A. I. Shaweesh, H. Matthews, A. Penington, Y. Fan, and J. G.
    Clement, 'Quantification of age-related changes in midsagittal
    facial profile using Fourier analysis: A longitudinal study on
    Japanese adult males' *Forensic Science International*, June 2019,
    volume 299, p. 239

19 Y. Cao, J. Yang, X. Zhu, et al., 'A Comparative In Vivo Study on
    Three Treatment Approaches to Applying Topical Botulinum
    Toxin A for Crow's Feet', *BioMed Research International*, July
    2018, volume 2018

20 N. Malek, D. Messinger, A. Yuan Lee Gao, E. Krumhuber,
    W. Mattson, R. Joober, K. Tabbane, I. C. Martinez-Trujillo,
    'Generalizing Duchenne to sad expressions with binocular
    rivalry and perception ratings', *Emotion*, March 2019, volume
    19, issue 2, pp. 234–241

21 R. D'souza, A. Kini, H. D'souza, N. Shetty, O. Shetty, 'Enhancing
    Facial Aesthetics with Muscle Retraining Exercises – A Review',
    Journal of Clinical and Diagnostic Research, August 2014, volume
    8, issue 8

22 Shaweesh, et. al, 'Quantification of age-related changes …,'

23 See www.nytimes.com/2006/07/27/books/27masl.html?_r=0

24 F. Tseng and H. Yu, 'Treatment of Horizontal Neck Wrinkles with
    Hyaluronic Acid Filler: A Retrospective Case Series' *Plastic and
    Reconstructive Surgery - Global Open*, August 2019, volume 7,
    p.2366

25 See www.businessinsider.com/dutch-town-traffic-lights-
    pavements-smartphone-addiction-2017-2?r=US&IR=T

26 See www.independent.co.uk/news/uk/home-news/office-posture-chair-hunch-back-doll-health-study-a9170316.html

27 See www.prnewswire.com/news-releases/national-sleep-survey-pulls-back-the-covers-on-how-we-doze-and-dream-184798691.html

28 Ibid.

29 Causing what is colloquially known as 'Cooper's droopers'.

30 See www.dermnetnz.org/topics/skin-phototype

31 See skincancer.org/skin-cancer-information/skin-cancer-facts

32 See www.theguardian.com/world/2016/mar/31/new-zealand-highest-rate-melanoma-skin-cancer

33 K. Mahendraraj, K. Sidhu, C. Lau, G. McRoy, R. Chamberlain and F. Smith, 'Malignant Melanoma in African–Americans', *Medicine*, April 2017, volume 96, issue 15

34 S. Rahrovan, F. Fanian, P. Mehryan, P. Humbert and A. Firooz, 'Male versus female skin: What dermatologists and cosmeticians should know', *International Journal of Women's Dermatology*, September 2018, volume 4, issue 3, pp. 122–130

35 See www.medicalnewstoday.com/articles/322887.php#4

36 See www.cosmopolitan.com/uk/beauty-hair/advice/a35197/drinking-water-skin-benefits

37 See www.thethirty.whowhatwear.com/why-does-coffee-make-me-tired

38 See www.nowpatient.com/how-can-gut-health-affect-your-skin-and-why

39 See www.theguardian.com/news/2018/mar/26/the-human-microbiome-why-our-microbes-could-be-key-to-our-health

40 See www.lifewaykefir.com/why-our-kefir-is-up-to-99-percent-lactose-free

41 Vollmer, et. al, 'Enhancing Skin Health: By Oral Administration of Natural Compounds and Minerals with Implications to the Dermal Microbiome' *International Journal of Molecular Sciences*, October 2018, volume 19, issue 10

42 Ibid.

43 Ibid.

44 See www.getoffyouracid.com/blogs/alkaline-info/the-truth-about-aging-vegetarians-you-might-not-like-this

45 See www.ewg.org/sunscreen/report/skin-cancer-on-the-rise

46 See /www.consumerreports.org/sunscreens/what-you-need-to-know-about-sunscreen-ingredients

47 See www.clearya.com/blog/safe-sunscreen-filters-according-to-science

48 M. A. Keen and I. Hassan, 'Vitamin E in dermatology', *Indian Dermatol Online Journal*, July–August 2016, volume 7, issue 4

49 See www.marieclaire.co.uk/beauty/skincare/face-peels-everything-you-need-to-know-253739

50 See www.instyle.com/beauty/skin/hydrafacial-treatment-facts

51 E. Caberlotto, et al., 'Effects of a skin-massaging device on the ex-vivo expression of human dermis proteins and in-vivo facial wrinkles', *PloS One*, March 2017, volume 12, issue 3

52 A common misconception exists around caffeine levels in flavoured or therapeutic tea blends. Jasmine and green tea, for example, have higher caffeine levels than coffee. Also, be aware that the terms 'decaffeinated' and 'alcohol-free' are used for marketing purposes. The former actually means reduced caffeine, not no caffeine. The latter typically contains 0.5 per cent alcohol.

53 See www.roguehealthandfitness.com/iron-causes-wrinkled-skin

54 See www.hemochromatosishelp.com/oxidation

About the Author

Dr Mike Dilkes has been a consultant Ear, Nose and Throat surgeon in London's Harley Street for more than 30 years. He is always at the forefront of new developments in his field and has innovated many new techniques over the years. Alexander Adams began his professional career as a clinical expert with GlaxoSmithKline. He has a talent for translating complex terminology into engaging formats, which anyone can understand and benefit from.

Stop Snoring the Easy Way will give you back control of your life, and explain why stopping snoring is not just desirable – it is essential.

STOP
SNORING

)))) ● ●(((

THE EASY WAY

How to breathe better, find relief and sleep well every night

DR MIKE DILKES & ALEXANDER ADAMS

Stop Allergies the Easy Way will help you understand your allergies and equip you with the tools to live the life you want, whatever the season.

STOP ALLERGIES

THE
EASY
WAY

The best way to
stop allergies from
ruining your life

**DR MIKE DILKES &
ALEXANDER ADAMS**